T0151429

Insomnia

Introduction

It's far into the night, but sleep won't come. You turn over. Perhaps a different position will quieten the mind. Or maybe the other side was better after all. Panic sets in. Not sleeping feels like a disaster. For very understandable reasons, our culture has arrived at extremely negative assessments of insomnia. It is a curse, to be overcome by art or science, by a sleeping pill, chamomile tea or sheep counting. But given how much time we may have to spend in the territory of sleeplessness, it is also worth attempting to map and understand the landscape – to learn to feel a little more at home with the idea of not being able to sleep and to view our insomniac hours as a challenging yet legitimate part of being human.

Our wakefulness can be interpreted as an artful revenge on the part of all the many deep, grand, significant and rich thoughts we did not properly attend to during the day. We can't sleep, in part, because we have so much unfinished thinking left to do.

The Danish painter Georg Friedrich Kersting hints at the virtues of the sleepless state. We can guess that it's very late for the man reading in his study; more conventional

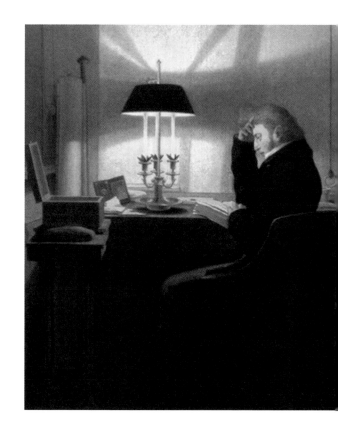

people have long ago turned in, but this man has stayed up, to finish a book, to think, to talk with a long-forgotten person: himself. Late at night is when big things may at last have a chance to happen in the mind. During the day, we are dutiful to others. At night we return to a bigger duty: to ourselves. Night is a corrective to the demands of the community. I may – in daytime hours – be a dentist or a maths teacher, a parent or a politician, but night is a reminder that I am also a nameless, limitless consciousness, a far more expansive, unanchored figure, of infinite possibilities and rare, disturbing, ambivalent, peculiar, visionary insights. The thoughts of night would sound weird to my mother, my friend, my boss, my child. These people need us to be a certain way. They cannot tolerate all our possibilities, and for some good reasons.

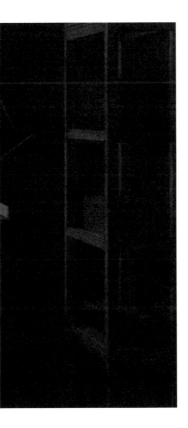

Georg Friedrich Kersting, *Man Reading by Lamplight*, 1814

We don't want to let them down; they have a right to benefit from our predictability. But their expectations can choke off important aspects of who we are. At night, with the window open and a clear sky above, it is just us and the universe – and for a time, we can take on a little of its boundlessness.

We are naturally inclined to want to be normal. Yet thanks to insomnia, we are granted a crucial encounter with our weirder, truer selves. We can learn of our own apparent strangeness. The daytime self is a misleading picture of what everyone is like. Insomnia is a gift – and a latent education.

Lots of books attempt to tell us how to sleep. This one will attempt to show us some of what happens while we can't sleep – so that we may feel less persecuted by, and alone with, our sleepless nights. It is a portrait of some of the more valuable, interesting and less-discussed things that happen in our minds at night, when we're supposed to be unconscious but are, in fact, more and more acutely conscious than at perhaps any other moment of our lives.

In our waking hours, for much of our lives, we are granted an unwarranted luxury: a sense that we are immortal. Our organs function normally, our joints give us no pains, we are focused on the next few financial quarters in the business. Dropping dead is the last thing on our minds.

But this is not the case in the early hours. Suddenly, there's an odd gnawing twinge in the stomach. It isn't anything major, and it might pass by tomorrow. But this might also be the start of a tumour that will fell us by New Year. Also, our chest feels a bit tight. When we breathe, there can sometimes be a sense of strain. There was an incident a little while back at the airport, running for the distant gate. Could it have been a heart attack, one of the quiet ones that passes largely undetected but tears fatefully at a valve? What about the slightly odd mole on one's back? Has it always been there or is it new, spreading aggressively and malignantly? Why can't we remember the name of that really nice colleague we worked with a few years back? Is reason beginning to crumble? This would be just the moment for a stroke that will leave us half-paralysed; paramedics will urgently wheel us along the A&E corridors on a trolley bed. We'll need to have our bottom wiped by a nurse and be fed with a tube coming out of our nose.

The sheer implausibility of being, and remaining, alive grows overwhelming. How is it possible that one can keep living, given everything that might go wrong? It isn't hypochondria any more, that macabre, almost fun state of mind you can adopt as an adolescent; this is a realistic assessment of the risks. It's the imagination correctly deployed.

This present ache or twinge might not announce the end – but something will happen. The abstract possibility of death turns, at night, into a concrete, decisive fact. Perhaps we'll fall off a ladder trying to get a suitcase out of a high-up cupboard and lie on the floor for eight hours with a broken neck, blood filling our lungs, before anyone finds our discoloured limp body. Or maybe we'll be lucky and it will be a quick aneurysm on the way back from a party celebrating a friend's birthday. Whatever it will be, it's getting closer. Others will be deeply distressed for a while; a few people will be sad even years later when they happen to think of us. But they'll cope. It won't matter to anyone the way it matters to us right now.

We're appalled and awed by the deep strangeness of being alive; it's so fundamentally improbable that the delicate web of our thoughts and feelings is being sustained by a bunch of pulpy, fragile organs. All our complicated ideas and lovely movements of the soul depend upon tiny mindless white blood corpuscles, oxygen molecules and the rhythmic spasms of the sinoatrial node. Why does the machine keep going? Why aren't we dead already?

The thoughts are horrific – and the full panic may go on for half an hour or more. But as we gradually grow used to the idea of being obliterated and forgotten, the thought of death sharpens our resolve: we have to do the important things while we can. We need to finish our work and dare to take up new initiatives. We need to forgive more. We can let a stupid comment pass; we can give up on a feud, even though the other wronged us.

The visceral knowledge of our approaching death renews our appreciation of existence. It's incredible to be able to hear a car accelerating in the distance; it's fascinating to have feet; the pillow feels so nice on our cheek; it will be lovely to look tomorrow at a tree or to hear a song or bite into a fig. We're brought back to a proper sense of the charm of things that ordinarily seem too slight to notice but that are close to why life is worth cherishing. The veil of jaded familiarity is pulled back – at least for a little while. A year starts to look like a huge privilege to have. A day when nothing much happens won't be boring; it will be a magnificent opportunity to

A We had managed to keep it, more or less, under control: using the busyness and reassuring familiarity of the working day to stop us from panicking. But now that there is nothing practical left to do, now that the world is eerie in its silence, the bank of anxieties hits us with new intensity.

If this were discovered, we could lose our job and our entire hard-won reputation; we might not be able to pay the mortgage or the rent; we might have to make a humiliating relocation; our partner might have an affair or leave us. Maybe the very stupid thing we did will be broadcast to the world; our worst moments will be made public – N acquaintances will look on us with anger and contempt; our attempts at self-defence will backfire; we'll never work again; our partner will forever be bitter and harsh. Our children will hate us. We'll be ruined and disgraced.

These thoughts don't come to us as theoretical possibilities or things that we suppose could possibly happen: at 3 a.m. they are what we have coming to us. After twenty minutes of ever-mounting tension, they build to a terrible high point of crisis: we are doomed, we have been moronic, our stupidity knows no bounds, our life is ghastly and pointless. It's unbearable. In desperation, we get out of bed and start to pace the room. Should we kill ourselves now? This isn't melodrama, just a sensible next step. Maybe we should go for a drive in the deserted streets? Or would we just be tempted to drive headlong off a bridge?

E We are like this for another half an hour, a portion of a private hell that no one will guess at when they see our normal, steady face in the morning. We are crying, clutching our head in our hands, banging our fists on the pillow, kneeling on the floor in a position of imploring prayer to a God we no longer believe in.

But then, just as it feels as if getting rid of ourselves is the only possible solution, another idea comes to mind. It doesn't deny any of the ghastly eventualities. It doesn't try to comfort us by telling us that everything will be OK. Instead, it looks at what will happen after the very worst has come to pass. It looks at the charred, wrecked landscape and asks us to see that a life of sorts could still be possible among the ruins.

It's true: there will be utter humiliation, everyone will mock, we'll lose the job; we won't have the money we were counting on. But, actually and rather remarkably, the sun will rise once more. We'll lose a leg, so to speak, but we will hobble on. We will be capable of living on far different terms from the ones we're currently used to. Millions of people do every day. It's not ideal but it can – almost – be all right.

After the disaster, there will be other things that come our way that we haven't thought of yet: new friendships, new ambitions, new satisfactions – less worldly, less materialistic, but genuine and properly rewarding. We can't tell how life will turn out exactly. We'll adjust, we'll manage. We'll find new reasons to be hopeful. There will – though it seems implausible now – be other days.

The way to reduce anxiety lies not in telling ourselves that the worst won't happen, but in exploring how even if the worst were to occur, we could find a way through. We need to make ourselves at home with the most horrific scenarios – and in so doing, we'll grasp that we're far less vulnerable to calamity than the spectres of the night insist.

4.

I've been so bad...

Our 3 a.m. self can privately admit that we've made many blunders...

During the day, we tend to brush away our more self-incriminating thoughts. When we face accusations from others, we angrily defend ourselves: it wasn't our fault; we weren't to blame; it's nothing to do with us. But now, in the night, we're more ready to admit to the inevitable truth: in many ways, of course, we have behaved appallingly and with great stupidity.

We're maybe not keen to go public with this, but our 3 a.m. self can privately admit that we've made many blunders. There are people we've hurt: there were kindly messages we didn't reply to. There are friendships we let slip for no big reason. There are secrets we've betrayed; people we've made fun of and belittled.

We've done some fairly disgusting things and made fools of ourselves: the awkward, fumbling attempts at sex; the lies we told; the cutting things we've said behind various people's backs.

We've been bad parents too. We should have spent more time with our children, we should have paid more attention to what they were trying to tell us and been more imaginative and agile in the questions we asked. We should have been nicer round the dinner table, and not let our own anxieties intrude so much.

We've been bad children too. We could have recognised the pressures our parents were under; there were times when we should have been more frank and others when we should have curbed our tongue. We should have taken many more chances to just let them know how we were getting on and shared the trivial things of life, which (we know) actually mean so much to them. We should have told them we loved them.

We have indeed been pretty awful. It feels terrible, but this is also a moment of growth in a very particular and very necessary direction: towards humility. We're dealing an important blow to our own self-righteousness. What makes people horrific is not so much that they make mistakes, but that they refuse to acknowledge with grace that they have made them.

In our night-time sorrow at our own errors, we're taking our modest place in the universal community of sinners. We realise how awful we can be – and in the process, become a little less so.

We were so slow to realise where our talents lay. We were so cautious in pressing ourselves forward. We took a slightly downbeat remark as outright rejection. We circled round a good idea but didn't push it hard enough. We were too loyal to a dead-end corporation or industry; we bowed to well-meaning but very bad advice; we believed in current acclaim rather than future success; we rushed too much, we hesitated too much; we didn't listen to our fears, we listened to them too much...

In the candour of the night, it's clear we've been fools in our careers. But our regrets and recriminations deserve to be placed in a larger perspective. Life inescapably confronts us with what can be described grandly yet accurately as an existential tragedy of choice. We are required to take major steps before we know enough about ourselves or the world. We are fated to rush, to steer blindly and to make moves that won't be right. We are entitled to a degree of compassion for our bad luck in having been born human, condemned by nature to navigate our hopes and ambitions from a position of inescapable ignorance.

Furthermore, we are so hard on ourselves chiefly because we know our own errors so intimately from the inside and know so little of the mistakes of others. Yet we can be sure that those we envy for their apparent good sense and sagacity are plagued by a raft of corrosive regrets of their own. Our deep consciousness of our blunders is something we have in common with pretty much everyone; it is in truth the most valuable material from which genuine, consoling friendships are built.

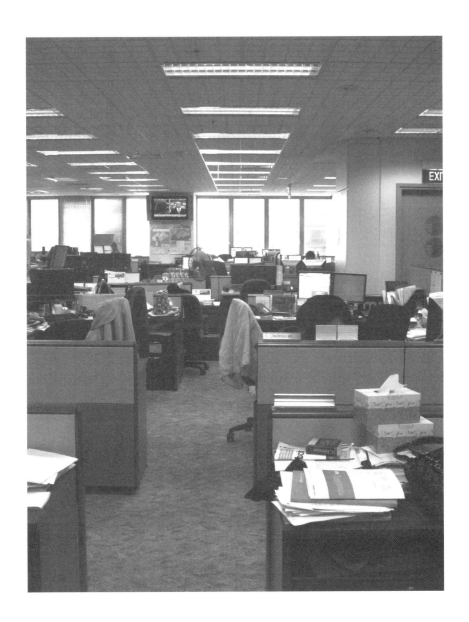

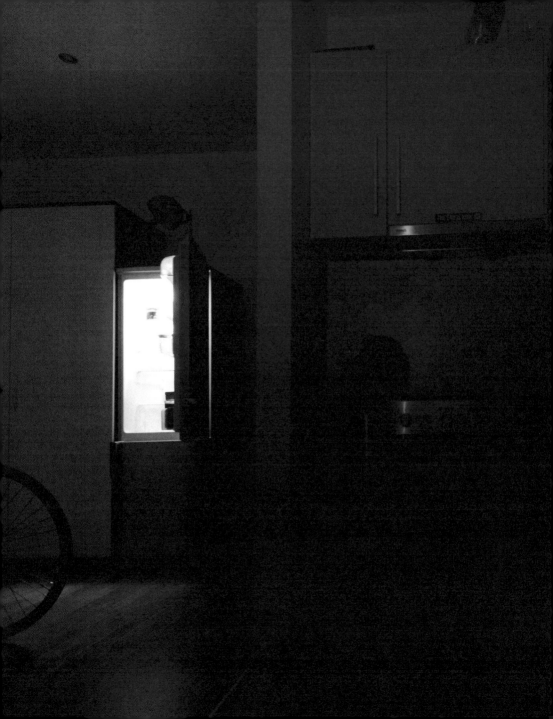

It feels odd to be here at this hour. We know the room so well, but at this strange time of night, it's like surprising an old friend in an unfamiliar part of town.

Everything is the way we remember it from the ordinary hours – and yet not quite. The room feels exceptionally quiet, a zone of deep tranquillity, relieved – for the time being – of all the usual friction, laughter and conversation.

The source of much art is the capacity to de-familiarise the things we know too well, so that we can learn to see their interest, beauty and fascination once more. A great painter can turn a blade of grass into an object of fascination. Now we're the artists of our own kitchens. We're newly confronting a familiar world and renewing our sense of its wonder.

There's a child's drawing on the fridge door: a fuzzy green dog with red ears or maybe a plane with grinning faces at each of its three windows – and only one wing. We can almost see the concentrated care with which it was done: the little tongue clamped between the teeth. They're seven years older now and hate to be associated with who they were then; they've become stand-offish, they don't want a piggyback

anymore and have stopped thinking we're wonderful guides to the world. The utter candour of the four-year-old has gone – it was so brief. The sweetest things are over in a flash. But they live on in a way – and just now we've found our way back to one example.

The kitchen tap emerges as a hugely bizarre, brilliant phenomenon: the terminal point of an incalculably vast system of tubes and cisterns, filtering stations, concrete pipes, pumping houses and reservoirs that expands into rivers, streams, drifting rain clouds, ocean currents and the prevailing winds of the upper atmosphere. We sip a mouthful or two and tip the rest down the plughole – via which a few droplets will eventually reunite with the cosmos.

We love the people who come in this kitchen more than they probably know, and more than we can normally convey. As we survey the photographs, the trinkets, the old pasta bowl near the fridge, the apron hanging from the door, the pile of books by the jar of oats, we realise that we have, after all, got so much to be grateful for – so much more than the day ever allows us to acknowledge.

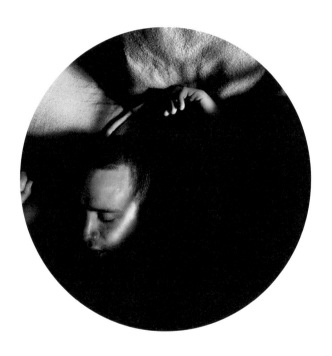

They have no idea
how carefully, and lovingly, we are
studying them. Their breathing is low
and even, with the occasional hesitation and
faint murmur. The eyelids are so delicate. Their hair
is disarranged. Briefly, a slight twitch animates the left
cheek. How deeply strange an ear is, seen from this
close. Lips that were earlier tense with annoyance are
sweetly parted; the brow that was creased in concentration
has relaxed. The troubling parts of who they are –
the parts that often demand most attention – are
silenced: they're not going to look at us sharply, ask
for anything or point out a problem at an
awkward moment. Now other sides to
them – always there but often
submerged – can

make it to the surface. We can recognise their generosity and their frankness, their sympathetic hesitation and their capacity for warm agreement. We can see again, perhaps, the person we first got together with; we can focus on the details we found so endearing: the specific slope of the cheek we longed to stroke, before we ever dared to; the corners of the mouth that flex delightfully when they try to hide their amusement.

A few hours ago they were doing the most ordinary things: reading the newspaper, chatting with their colleagues, wondering how much salt to add to a dish. Now we wonder what landscape of emotions and memories they are travelling in. They might be taken up with themes that date from the long period before we knew them. They might be chasing the dog they had as a child, surfing at a beach far away with friends we've never met, searching for something in their childhood bedroom, which we've never seen – or revisiting the unique passions that tied them to a former lover. In the morning they won't be able to tell us and we'll never find out. We're encountering the profound fact that, however well we think we know them, we will only ever meet a little of who they fully are. The immensity of their inner life, expanded across time, will always be closed to us, not out of sly secretiveness or ill-will but for a more moving and profound reason: the core human inability to turn our most intimate experiences into meaningful words.

At this moment we feel more pity and tenderness towards them than we have for a very long time. It's not that we've forgotten the ways they've frustrated us. It's rather that our resentment and disappointment have been united with a correct and awe-inspiring sense of their beauty, intelligence and astonishing kindness in agreeing to spend their lives with us.

We must, somehow, find a way to mention a little of this to them in the morning.

...the cheek we longed...
...that flex delightfully when they...
...y were doing the most ordinary things:
...r colleagues, wondering how much salt to ad...
...dscape of emotions and memories they are travell...
...ith themes that date from the long period before we...
...sing the dog they had as a child, surfing at a beach far a...
...met, searching for something in their childhood bedroo...
...or revisiting the unique passions that tied them to a form...
...y won't be able to tell us and we'll never find out. We'...
...fact that, however well we think we know them, we wi...
...hey fully are. The immensity of their inner life, expa...
...sed to us, not out of sly secretiveness or ill-will bu...
...n: the core human inability to turn our mos...
...s. At this moment we feel more pit...
...y long time. It's not that...

We have quite a few of them, we realise, as we lie unable to sleep. There's a very long roll-call of people who've been mean, annoying, boring, tactless, graceless or offensively stupid around us. Humanity is almost universally rotten. In this mood, we feel like Noah before he built the ark: asked by God to find ten decent people on earth, he had to report back that, in fact, there weren't any, besides himself and his close family. When we consider all the bullies, the braggarts, the selfish, the self-righteous, the naive, the slimy, the brutish, the brash, the shallow, the pompous, the cold, the greedy, the freeloaders and the exploiters of others, we can sympathise with the plan of flooding the earth and starting again.

But once we've reached the climax of bitterness there's a very different mood that can begin to make itself felt. Maybe it starts with ourselves: in our own way we are pretty awful and yet at our core, we know we're nice enough. We mean well. It's true we blunder, we show off, we say the wrong things... but we know the fuller story. We're trying to cope as best we can. We're harried and put upon and burdened by difficulties we didn't choose. We deserve tenderness rather than scorn, even though our failings are very real.

And then we broaden the circle. Others are like this too. Everyone has been

R E
S E N T

damaged by things they didn't choose; they're struggling, frail, and unfortunate in ways we'll never know. Perhaps the elegantly attired individual hasn't spoken to their daughter for three years and they know it's their fault and they don't know how to put it right. The bully was bullied; the boaster is in desperate recoil from past humiliations. And every one of these is touched – at times when we're not around to look – by beauty and grace. They've felt shame, they've longed for love, they've wanted to be understood and cherished; they've cried at certain musical phrases, they've delighted in a fresh summer morning. It's true they're awful, but it's nothing like the whole truth.

We're viewing a world of unmerited pain and thus we come alive to the universal need for kindness. We are all hopelessly fragile, proud, weak creatures yearning for redemption and forgiveness. In our hearts, a great, majestic tide of compassion rises to meet every unknown sorrow in the world. Without anyone being there to observe it, we start to learn to love.

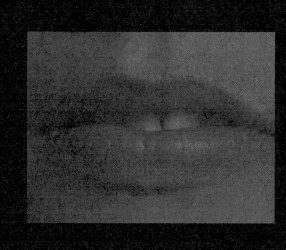

Imaginary speeches

What we say in reality to other people is only a fraction of what we think of saying to them in our heads. Most of what we really want to express is kept back for private, imaginary speeches we give inside our minds, very often in the middle of our sleepless nights.

These speeches aren't dress rehearsals for a daytime delivery. The intended audiences may be dead or living elsewhere, or they would be incapable of listening to us in any case. But the deeply private, night-time act of rehearsal has a legitimacy all of its own. Simply ordering and refining what we'd like to say contains many of the benefits of real expression. We should honour the legitimacy of imaginary speeches.

Here are some of the speeches we might deliver in the darkness:

You mean so much to me. I know how hard it's been for you. If I don't see you as much as I should, it's not out of coldness, but out of an intensity of feeling I'm sometimes afraid of. You gave me life and more than that, you taught me everything I know about decency. I know I pushed you away as I grew up. Once I called you boring and I regret it to this day. I loved it when I was off school and could stay with you alone. I remember the way you'd make me a boiled egg and bring it to me in bed or wrap me up warmly on the sofa and let me watch TV. I remember the way you stroked my hair forward and held me close to you. I'm so sorry I let you down. I love you so much.

You accused me of indifference, but all I've ever wanted to do was gain your love. When you shouted at me when I was little, I wanted to cry: it wasn't because I resented you, but because I was so sorry for upsetting you. I wanted you to be proud of me. I don't think you know how much you've influenced me and how often I think of you. So much of what I do has you as its intended audience. I'm not really cold and not properly distant. I just don't know how to begin to be your friend.

It was so unpleasant sometimes. I can't forget how it was during the Berlin meeting. But it can't be the whole story. I don't blame you: I didn't really have the chance to show you the right sides of me. I was still so immature. With different luck, we could have been friends – if we'd bumped into each other on holiday or if we'd met a few years later. Other people found you a bit intimidating and I did too – but for me it was the kind of intimidation that comes when you admire someone but don't know if they'll admire you back. I think of you more than you could possibly imagine. Once I had a dream about you. Recently I was changing flights at Frankfurt and I thought I saw you in the distance. It would be good to run into you somewhere.

It was so nice talking to
you at the reception. I
was very excited when
you suggested going on
somewhere for a drink.
There was a point when
we were laughing and you
leaned your head towards
me and whispered
something funny. It was
a lovely conspiratorial
moment; the two of us
together against the
general idiocy of everyone
else. I'm sorry I suddenly
seemed cold and just
went home. I wish we
could have exchanged
numbers. There was
a lot going on in my
life and maybe I was
frightened that this could
be serious and I wasn't
ready for it. It's mad, but
I think of you a lot still.
In my head you are still
someone central: you're
in all the chapters of the
autobiography of the life I
never led.

I know it's fashionable
to hate you and I admit
there are things on
which we don't see eye
to eye. But it's not the
differences that interest
me. I can just about
imagine the pressures
you are under and how
different it all looks to
you from the way it does
to your critics. I'm going
to say it: I wish I could
be your friend. I feel I
could help you on certain
points. I wish you were
able to tell me what's
on your mind and share
a few of your troubles.
There are times when
I'd love you to be a touch
bolder or a little softer
and sweeter – and I think
you could be if you knew
a friend was with you.
I wish you could ring
me up at night and talk
through the news of the
day and what's really
going on behind the
headlines. You could

share your sorrows
and worries with me; we
could mull over the needs
of the country; you could
confide your hopes in
me. We can't make things
perfect, but together we
could maybe get a few
wiser nudges to work.
I wish we were going out
to dinner tomorrow, just
the two of us.

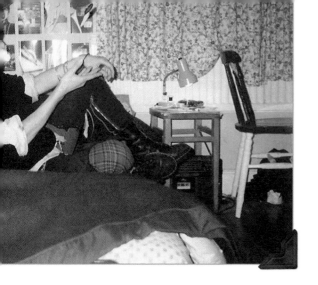

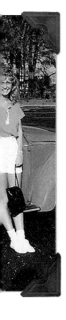

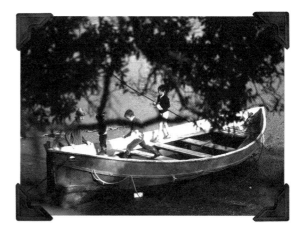

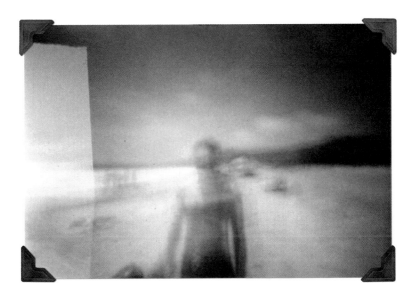

There is so much material in our minds
that we seldom visit in our waking hours.
We have, surprisingly, forgotten almost
nothing that we ever lived through. We just
need the right amount of calm to bring it
to the surface. An inner photographer has
taken shots of pretty much everything we
experienced: the highlands of Scotland
we went to when we were ten; the store
room in our grandmother's house on
the archipelago; the light on a Sunday
evening as we drove home from a party
shortly after our twentieth birthday.

These things rarely come to mind in the press of the working day, but sometimes – when we can't sleep – we realise that it is all still there and we find ourselves travelling back through images and scenes we had not suspected had survived with such clarity. The memories are not necessarily significant in and of themselves, but they are vivid and overwhelming in their immediacy, like the most beautiful frame of a film. For example: we are seven again. It is a Saturday morning; the sun is shining through the bedroom curtains; the wallpaper has big pink and blue flowers. We are waiting for everyone to wake up and are on the floor, designing a game on a large sheet of paper. The mood is serene and focused and filled with hope. Or, we are in New York for the first time. We must be thirty. It is an intensely warm, almost tropical, evening and we wander the streets of Lower Manhattan; we can recall the pavements, the restaurants, the shape of the buildings. We go into a shoe repair store and talk a little to the owner. We can remember the smell of leather and polish. Or five years ago, we are on a trip to Asia: we are coming into Singapore at night. We have a window seat and can see a long line of lights of tankers and container ships and perhaps some small fishing vessels too. Gazing down, the modern world looks majestic and calm, beautiful and ordered. In the full range of our memories we're bigger than we suppose. At some point or other across our lives we've met so much – and though it has receded deep into the cavities of the mind, it can re-emerge with the right meditative night-time frame of mind.

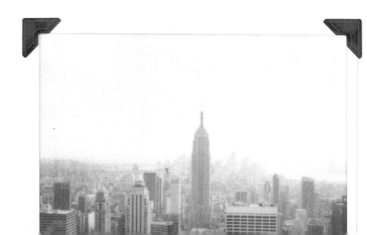

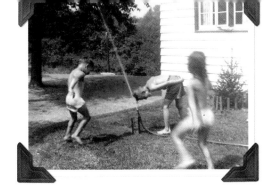

Little attention normally gets paid to our sensory memories. We don't engineer regular encounters with them. We may feel we have to dismiss them as 'daydreaming' or 'thinking about nothing'. But in our neglect of our memories, we are spoilt children, who squeeze only a portion of the pleasure from experiences and then toss them aside to seek new thrills. Part of why we feel the need for so many new experiences may simply be that we are so bad at absorbing the ones we have had.

When we can't sleep, we should always think of going on Memory Journeys. Our experiences have not disappeared, just because they are no longer unfolding right in front of our eyes. We can remain in touch with so much of what made them pleasurable simply through the art of evocation. We talk endlessly of virtual reality. Yet we don't need gadgets. We have the finest virtual reality machines already in our own heads. We can – right now – shut our eyes and travel into, and linger amongst, the very best and most consoling bits of our past.

It is not surprising if, in most of our minds, there is a constant static hum of worry around the future. There are so many things we have to schedule, and do, every single day: we haven't replied to that email from a friend of a friend; there's a new point that has to be squeezed into the report; we need to change the time of the dental appointment for next week; we have to talk a client through a problem that's come up with a project; we need to think about getting someone a birthday present; the second bulb over the dining table needs to be replaced; the car has to be collected from the garage; we have to visit our grandmother. Then we have to think of timings: the plane goes at 3.15 so we'll need to be at the airport around two, which means we'll have to leave at one – but it depends on the traffic – so maybe ten to one would be better; so we'll have to get out of the meeting by 12.45 and let a couple of people know that we'd best discuss the main item earlier – it shouldn't be a problem (though we should have told them a few days ago); and we should phone our mother at some point between breakfast and the first meeting; we must make the payment for the electricity bill and have to drop a couple of things off at the dry cleaners ahead of the Milan trip. The mind is, by this point, understandably, red-hot with panic – and the possibility of sleep seems ever further away.

It is beautifully and almost insultingly simple to think that what we most urgently need to do at this point is to switch on a bedside light, get a piece of paper and a pen out and start to make a list. Far from being a humble or trivial activity, the drawing up of lists constitutes one of the most incisive, grand and relevant gestures we can ever make to correct the natural failings of our minds. These minds did not evolve to juggle thirty different streams of responsibility a day. Our lists are embodiments of what civilisation can do to improve on raw nature.

The function of a list isn't to magically reduce the number of things we have to do. It's to control the mind. Much of anxiety is about the fear of forgetting. It's as if each task has its own determined, nervous advocate in our brains who continually questions whether we have kept their singular priority in our mind. With inquisitorial aggression, they ask: 'Have you forgotten...? What time do you plan to get to...?' Every few moments, we need to calm them down and answer that their item remains on our agenda, and that is enough to ensure we will never sleep.

But once we've physically written an item down we can – in effect – close off the nagging voice. We can point them to our list and prove that we've got things in hand: yes, we've remembered: look, it's written down, as clear as day.

Spread out on a list, our lives look more manageable. What had seemed like an infinity of tasks turns out to be 'only' two dozen. We can draw little arrows about what needs to be done in what order. We can cross off items that don't strictly need to be conquered in the next twenty-four hours. We can see the month ahead in a glance. A list is such a modest thing, we forget what important work it does for us. We cannot hold all our lives in our own minds at once. We should regularly let a piece of paper and some bullet points perform their distinctive magic.

The end of the world

We check the time on our phone – it's 3.47 a.m. – and then immediately scan the news. We're lying in the dark, still half asleep, looking at a tiny glowing screen and slowly we're realising that, this time, it might really be the end: the world really could fall apart.

During the day, things had seemed a bit more solid. We knew there were risks but we were preoccupied with what was immediately in front of us: we needed to finish a bit of work, the carpet in the hallway was starting to look threadbare, we had to remember to buy some more eggs.

But now we give ourselves over to the future of our species and the verdict is not good at all: a few unbalanced people could blow us all sky high in a fit of temper, unstoppable plagues could spread around the world in days, economic catastrophe could destroy the whole system. We grow vibrantly alive to the tragic potential that's always lurking in the human project.

We might be seeing the end of civilisation just as the Romans did: then, roads that had been maintained for centuries fell into total disrepair; aqueducts, constructed with astonishing ingenuity, ran dry; barbarians who once inhabited unimaginably remote forests looted nearby towns and cities; money stopped circulating; trade collapsed; an educated society became largely illiterate. In the deep night, we admit a version of this could happen again. There's no logic of history or innate communal wisdom that ensures it won't. Humanity doesn't have a guaranteed progressive destiny. And this isn't merely an intellectual speculation. We're looking – via our phone – at an entirely real vision of the future.

With such thoughts in mind, what is the good of tomorrow? How can we respond with a conventionally cheery 'fine' when people ask how we're doing? It feels impossible to reconcile the hysterical visions of our insomniac selves with the sensible requirements of our daytime existence.

And yet we can; we are – remarkably – creatures who can contemplate the ultimate ruin of the world and yet still cheerily head off to work tomorrow.

We are natural geniuses at integration: we can have a degree of cosmic gloom and, at the same time, a robust, pragmatic enthusiasm for the local demands and pleasures of our days. The species may die out – but we should tuck in the corners of the sheets when we make the bed; people we loathe and fear may dominate the world – but do these shoes go OK with this jacket? We can contemplate the grand-scale darkness – and still sensibly get on with the sober tasks of the day ahead.

In the night, a thought about our childhood comes to mind: the bedroom we had when we were nine; a long car trip staring out the back-seat window; a stuffed bear that used to keep us company in bed. And the memories grow out from there: we used to get excited because we were going to have fish fingers for lunch; we looked forward all week to the next episode of a favourite television programme and hummed the title music in the bath. In the sandpit we could scoop tunnels through cold damp sand; we liked pretending to be a rabbit or an elephant; we loved crawling under our bed; there was a story about a bird with a broken wing that used to make us cry; we saved up some pocket money and bought a kite; we spent ages drawing pictures of a place called 'mouseland'. We envied a friend who had a spacesuit with a helmet and a visor that flipped up and down. There was a lovely evening when we visited some friends of our parents in the country and we played with their children in a wild garden until it got so dark we could hardly see. Not everything was lovely, of course; but in this insomniac night-time mood we're more alive to the sweeter moments.

We were so innocent back then. Money never entered our thoughts except in comically small amounts; sex sounded alien and essentially uninteresting; a crisis meant not remembering the answer to 7×8, or leaving our sports top at home. By contrast the adult world looks so anxious and so depraved. The comparison can feel very sad. It's as if growing up has meant the hardening and coarsening of a self that used to be simple and delicate; there's been a loss of beauty and of the power to be moved and excited by small things.

And yet, the fact is, we've not truly lost the childhood parts of ourselves. They are still speaking to us in our thoughts. We can re-find a degree of innocence.

Without surrendering the advances of adulthood we can keep faith with who we once were. We can be enchanted by a hedgehog and keep an eye on the stock market indices; we can get on in a legal career and remember the thrill of hide-and-seek. Ideally we should inject what we knew when we were small – the sweetness of a game, the joy of being naughty, the delight of pretending – into the tasks of adult life.

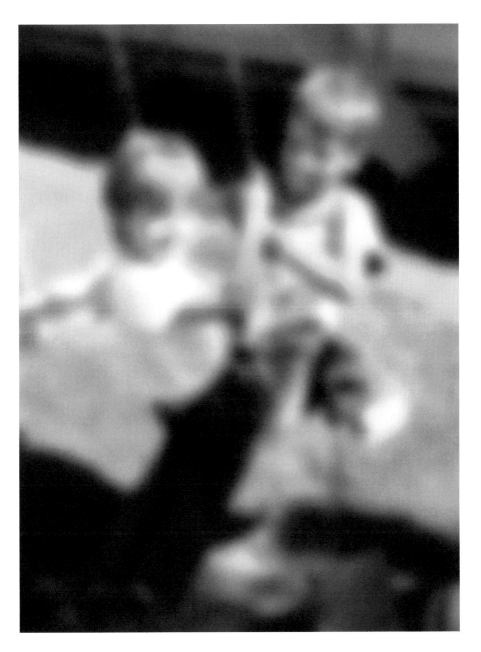

14.

On Reading

Maybe reading for a bit will tire the mind and induce us finally to sleep. So we pick up a novel. We've heard good things about it. And we've read countless stories in our time. But at this moment – with our heads filled with our own night thoughts – the novel feels like hard work. The author is going to great lengths to get us interested in the life of someone living in Edinburgh in the 1930s; it's raining a lot and their car breaks down; they've got a friend in Budapest who is pregnant; there's a robbery at a department store. There's a reference to Dundas Street and we flick back thirty pages and realise that's where the main character's sister used to live. There's a retired engineer with very bushy eyebrows who must be important in some way we don't know yet.

Immense effort and intelligence are being devoted to exploring the existence of a fictional individual. No-one, we realise, has ever looked at our life – our habits, our friends, our past, our dilemmas and problems – with such sustained curiosity or in such detail. In this book, there are pithy insights, clever summations, striking observations and astute analyses, but all for the sake of the workings of the mind of someone else, who's not really very much like us. It's a familiar situation we've just taken for granted. But now it hits us: we're reading the wrong book. What we should really be doing is reading a book about us – written with the same elegance and wisdom, but placing the raw material of our life in a lucid order, selecting and joining up diverse events and turning them into a coherent story.

Maybe reading for a bit will tire the mind and induce us finally to sleep.

So we pick up a novel...

What we really crave is for someone to make loving sense of us and write it all down in crisply phrased sentences. Our reading of someone else's novel is as if we went to the doctor and they made a very accurate diagnosis of someone else's earache, or if a financial advisor went to great lengths to present us with a solution to the money troubles of a stranger, from which we could at best extract the occasional fleeting hint of what might possibly be useful in our own case.

Frankenstein
Mary Shelley

Alice's Adventures in Wonderland
Lewis Carroll

The House of Sleep
Jonathan Coe

The Iliad
Homer

A Midsummer Night's Dream
Shakespeare

The Interpretation of Dreams
Sigmund Freud

Wuthering Heights
Emily Brontë

In the 1690s, one of the greatest of French writers, François Fénelon, was appointed tutor to the young Duke of Burgundy. To assist with his education, Fénelon wrote a long and fascinating novel called *The Adventures of Telemachus* in which the Duke, lightly disguised, was the central character. The problems the character in the novel faces were exactly the problems the Duke was actually facing; the strengths and weaknesses of the central character – carefully understood by the writer – were his. It sounded like the rarest and most cultivated luxury to have someone write a novel about you. But in fact it is one that we can in principle provide for ourselves.

We don't need to give up our jobs and become writers, because this book of ourselves is one we're writing already; we're at work on it in the early hours, when we can't sleep, when we daydream, make plans, go over the past – and give ourselves over to retelling, as best we can, what has really happened to us and what it all could mean.

Insomnia provides us with the time to ask ourselves some of the large questions that we don't usually get round to during the day. It's akin to how a management team might head out of the office for a few hours in order to think through the bigger, underlying strategic issues of the business that they wouldn't otherwise find the time to consider properly.

Our agenda of issues, for discussion with ourselves, might ideally be built around some of the following enquiries:

What would I like to change about myself?

_____

_____

_____

_____

_____

_____

_____

Without being harsh on our existing selves, we're getting interested in the fact that the way we are right now isn't completely fixed: there's a degree of flexibility – and a need for improvement.

What would I like to achieve?

_____

_____

We're not making a fantasy wish-list, untethered to the reality of life; we're exploring the borderline territory between a frank assessment of our own capacities and our larger hopes and ambitions: the things we might just be able to pull off, if we set about them in the right way. Sometimes we'll be expanding on an existing plan – what if we pushed it harder, did it on a bigger scale? At other points we'll be taking an ideal and slimming it down, paring it back to more manageable proportions.

How would I like to be around people I love?

| What do I regret? |

_____

_____

_____

_____

_____

_____

_____

Often, sadly, the people we're closest to only get to see a limited version of who we are. We can be quite witty with our friends – but that's not often on show at home. We have a tendency, maybe, to harbour resentments: we're still hurt by something they did last year; we'd like to be lighter and more focused on the possibilities of the future. We could let them know more often how much they mean to us; we could be a touch more patient; we could share a little more of our inner life.

Regrets aren't just a chance to beat ourselves up. A frank assessment of how we have let ourselves and others down becomes a map for future improvement.

The questions are calming not because they provide neat solutions but because just by asking them we start to clarify some of the muddled zones of our minds. We're not merely lying pointlessly in bed; we're mapping our own minds.

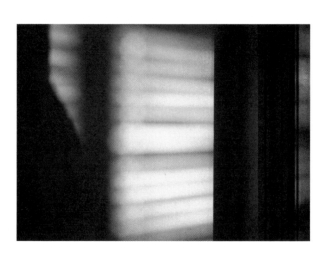

The standard habit of the mind is to take careful note of what's not right in our lives and our environment. Any irritation, however small, announces itself loudly in our brains. It's probably a legacy of evolution. We're the descendants of those who worried: the ones who noticed a slight movement in the grass and assumed the presence of a snake; the ones who in the warm days of summer fretted about what they'd eat in winter.

But a consequence is that the balance of the day, and of our lives, is not accurately drawn up. We are experts at filling in the debit side – the list of everything that went wrong, that isn't entirely OK and that might go badly in the future. But we're haphazard and negligent when it comes to the credit side: the register of what was nice and pleasant and interesting, and the list of all the things that didn't go wrong. Our brains gloss over the modest positives – because from the extreme perspective of keeping us alive they don't require urgent attention. Yet if we don't properly recognise them we're getting a badly distorted picture of our lives. We feel things are much worse than they really are. It takes a nudge from the will to redirect our attention and consciously identify what there is to be grateful for.

Night-time allows us to take stock: the car didn't break down; we turned a tap and hot water emerged; we're in good health. Sometimes the children are kind. Our partner is – at points – extremely generous. It's been quite warm lately. Yesterday, we were happy all afternoon. We're quite enjoying our work at the moment.

We're not forgetting our ambitions or pretending that everything good in life is simple and inexpensive. But the case for striving is already well made: we're not on the cusp of forgetting the appeal of material success or a new house. It's the case for the less obvious things we need to remind ourselves of. In the darkness, we can remember what we have to be grateful for.

17.

Someone once sang you to sleep

You're alone now with your wakeful thoughts. But long ago, another person took care to ease you towards sleep. They helped you sip a warm drink. They tucked you up, leaving a soothing fold of sheet just under your nose; they dimmed the lights. They stroked your cheek and ear with the back of their fingers. They read you a story, their voice gradually quietening as they saw your eyes start to close. They sang you a song – maybe the same one someone sang to them at bedtime in the mythical time when they were little. They held you and whispered the sweetest secret names. They kissed your forehead one last time, and brushed your hair away from your face with the gentlest touch; they tiptoed out of your room, leaving the door open just a fraction so that a little light would still come in from the hall.

Life is very imperfect but this person did something wonderful – they founded an essential premise in your soul: you can be loved apart from your achievements and merits, you can be precious to another person just because you exist. And this opens the strangest of possibilities: your own capacity to be generously tender to another, even when they don't much deserve it. You may often feel quite far from love but, as you remember the warmest moments of childhood, you realise again how much you want and need it.

They   a song   to

    you   them

sang   someone   at

    maybe   sang   bedtime

      one

    the

   the

in   time   little

    when   were

mythical

    they

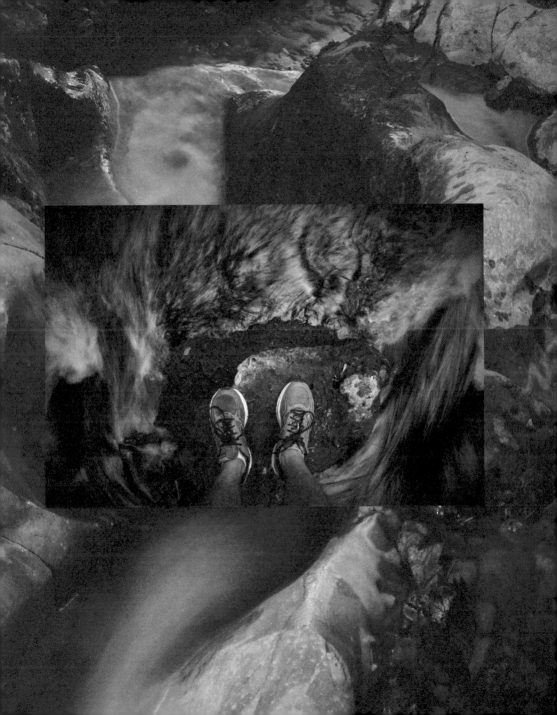

Often, as we emerge from sleep in the middle of the night, there's a dream still vivid and intact in our minds. But even as we try to remember what it was about, it starts to fade: the recollection is so delicate it can't survive being handled by our conscious minds. Only a few odd images and fragments remain: we were going down a crowded escalator; there was a guard with a gun; there was a ploughed field; we were saying something crucial to the Prime Minister – who looked like someone in our class when we were nine. But, even as the surrounding details and the intricacies of the storyline dissolve, there's a vague afterglow: the dream was dramatic, intense and emotionally rich; it was filled with ideas and insights, though it's hard now to say what they were.

Generally, we might not think of ourselves as being particularly creative – but at night our brains reveal a very different potential. It's as if we have an elaborate film studio located inside our heads. A genius director and a hugely inventive team of writers produce new features for us every night. They've taken us to Spain but recreated a street so it looks like Chicago; they've hired a former colleague for the role of an astronaut; they've taken over the family home of the first person we went out with and inserted a swimming pool in the bathroom; they've summoned a long-dead grandmother back to life to be the passenger in a taxi we're driving. They've shot scenes from surprising angles; they've interwoven fantastically elaborate and gripping plot-lines. They've studied every phase of our life and investigated every detail of our emotional history. And every night they cast us as the lead actor.

A dream is often a container for insights we didn't know we had: we hadn't realised that the holiday we went on when we were seven still meant so much to us (the studio has lovingly recreated the sand dunes on the beach and found again the blue bucket we used for making sandcastles); we'd not properly grasped how frightened we are of being abandoned by a particular friend (in the dream it didn't occur to them that we couldn't ski and they raced off down the mountain without us).

Our dream life – even if we recall only a tiny portion of it – reveals us as much more complex, imaginative and strange beings than we purport to be during our waking hours. There's so much going on in our heads – and no-one else will really know or care very much about it. Our dreams carry a rightly astonishing implication: everyone is like this on the inside. The rather dull-looking individual who works in the next office, the old lady with the large handbag we saw in the street, the genial TV host – each one contains within them a vastly elaborate and imaginative dream-world that may be greatly at odds with their outer demeanour, but that (if only we could access it) would offer a deeper and more accurate guide to who they truly are.

When we dream it's as if our brain is hinting to us: 'I'm a poet, I'm a visionary, I'm capable of anything. I'm Cecil B. DeMille – so use me, let me out, take me with you when you go to work, when you're writing a marketing email, when you talk to your child, when you're having dinner with your partner. Don't let me out only at night.' Our dreams hint that our minds could be capable of so much more than we allow them to do in the day.

As children, when someone asked our age, we might have said 'I'm four and a half'. We didn't want anyone to think we were only four. A few months had taken us far beyond what we had been before. And the huge dignity of turning five still seemed very far away. We were conscious, that is, of the rapidity and intensity of our development and we wanted to signal this to others and ourselves in the clearest way we could – with a number.

It would sound comic or a touch mad for an adult to say proudly: 'I'm twenty-five and a half' or 'forty-one and three quarters' – because, without particularly noticing, we've drifted away from the notion that adults, too, are engaged in constant evolutions. But in truth we may have grown significantly over the last six months or the previous week. There won't be a simple outward measure: we're no taller, we've not boosted our seniority at work and received a new title to confirm our growth to the world. And what external changes there are may offer no clues to the kind of progress we've actually made: a receding hairline doesn't indicate that we've come to a new understanding of our mother; a deepening wrinkle around the eye can't show our acquaintances that we've constructively altered our ideas about what success means.

A lot of what we learn happens at night. We may have, over a sleepless night, re-thought our attitude to money or come to an important insight about family life. We may have made a momentous step in self-forgiveness or resolved one of the riddles of our partner's character. Our evolution often proceeds when we can't sleep and our mind is free enough – and has enough time – to consider what's really going on in our lives.

These quiet, but very real, milestones don't get marked. We're not given a cake or a present to mark the special occasion. We're not congratulated by others and viewed with enhanced respect. At school we pass through the various years of study in a very clear way: we're tested and examined to determine what we've learned. We get graded on our attainments. We learn just as much, or more, in the school of night, but without the formal charting of our progress.

We harbour a muffled demand that our own evolution should be properly recognised by others. It's the adult version of the way a thirteen-year-old bristles at the idea that someone thinks they are still twelve. We tend not to love our birthdays so much as we get older, because the mere passing of years isn't any longer a proper index of how we're changing. We find it tricky to put into words how we've changed and others aren't necessarily very eager to hear much about it.

In an ideal, utopian world our inner progress would be clearly charted; we'd be warmly congratulated by our friends on the way we'd evolved in our attitude to money or on the impressive way we'd re-thought our ideas of what a holiday should be like. In the meantime, we should take pride in our ongoing efforts to learn; in the way we are dutiful students of the school of night.

SO
WHAT
IF
I DON'T
SLEEP...

We haven't slept much and it will soon be time to start the day. There's a moment of panic: we're going to be so tired, we'll be dragging ourselves through all the things we have to do.

But we can almost feel proud of our sleeplessness. We've accomplished so much. We've journeyed through our past; we've faced our own death, we've seen the end of the world, we've spoken with the dead; we've visited the remote regions of our own minds and come to know better the parts of ourselves that inhabit them; we've maybe made peace with an enemy and re-found a lost love, and redrawn the balance of our ambitions and our failings. We've pieced together what we think, we've acknowledged and investigated our fears.

It's only been a few hours but an immense amount has happened to us. Our tiredness will have the pleasing, slightly heroic quality that comes after finishing a big task. The day won't be perfect. It will be wrong in all the familiar ways. But we'll be meeting it from a different starting point with a little more wisdom and compassion, both for others and for ourselves. Perhaps we'll be able to get to bed early this evening. And it won't be so bad when, as is bound to happen on certain future nights, we find ourselves sleepless again.

Published in 2019 by The School of Life
First published in the USA in 2019
70 Marchmont Street, London, WC1N 1AB

Printed in Latvia by Livonia

A proportion of this book has appeared online at
www.theschooloflife.com/thebookoflife

The School of Life is a resource for helping us
understand ourselves, for improving our relationships,
our careers and our social lives – as well as for helping
us find calm and get more out of our leisure hours.
We do this through creating films, workshops, books
and gifts.

www.theschooloflife.com

10 9 8 7 6 5 4 3

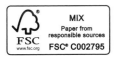

Picture credits:
Man Reading by Lamplight, Georg Friedrich Kersting,
1814. *The office in Singapore*, Craige Moore, Flickr.
Fridge, Janels Katlaps, Flickr. *Watching someone sleeping*,
Cia de Photo, Flickr. *Barons Court haircut*, wetwebwork,
Flickr. *At Play*, Sid Mosdell, Flickr. *Dreams*, katieg93,
Flickr. *I want to wake up in a city, That doesn't
sleep*, Sasha Kargaltsev, Flickr. *Hoser!*, Susan, Flickr.
*Caribbean Gulf Petroleum Explosion – American
Airlines*, Tomás Del Coro, Flickr. *Swing*, Michelle
Hofstrand, Flickr. *Day 136: Evening Light*, Tom Small,
Flickr.

The School of Life is a global organisation helping people lead more fulfilled lives. It is a resource for helping us understand ourselves, for improving our relationships, our careers and our social lives – as well as for helping us find calm and get more out of our leisure hours. We do this through films, workshops, books, gifts and community. You can find us online, in stores and in welcoming spaces around the globe.

THESCHOOLOFLIFE.COM

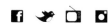